# Moments that Made Us

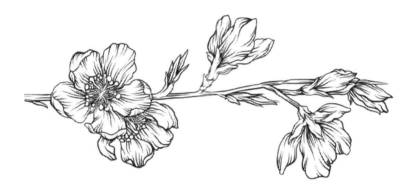

## Joan Cruz

# DEDICATION

For nurses.

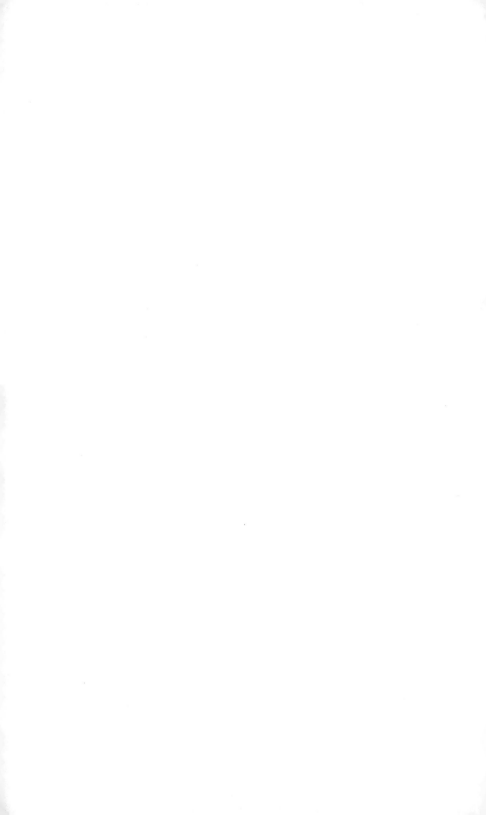

# CONTENTS

# ACKNOWLEDGMENTS

To my friends, who never doubted the writer in me.

To my sister, who I am so lucky to have in this life.

To my dad, who knew I was a writer before anyone did.

And to Jan, who always made sure my words were seen and adored.

"Sometimes I inspire my patients; more often they inspire me." —Unknown

"I attribute my success to this; I never gave nor took any excuse." —Florence Nightingale

"The meaning of life is to find your gift. The purpose of life is to give it away."
—William Shakespeare

# I.
## Nursing is an art

## Legacy

We sprung from a woman's courage,
a caring heart and vision so clear
With wise words, she had taught us,
"How very little can be done under the spirit of fear."
So that during times of turmoil,
we can rise to be who we need to be
Unseen heroes that are nurses,
Nightingale's living legacy.

# Incoming

we were fifteen hours into the air
    when the body of
the airplane started its dive back to Earth.
every little lunge felt in my stomach,
each inch closer to the ground,
    a mile away from the familiar.

my mind eclipsed with a headache but
my gut fluttered with the dawn
    of a new beginning;
fresh as the cool April day that received us-
clear and sunny, the sky almost gushed
    welcome.
the fourteen-degree air seeped through fabric
and dug deep into my spine,
like I have never known before.

around the corner, a solitary tree danced,
beckoned into glorious unfurling,
pink as the over-sized luggage
stuffed with my life at the seams.

    you will get used to the cold.
you will learn to soothe the distance
between you and where you came from,
much like how I dwelled in the comfort
of Sinigang cooked in someone else's pot
for my first dinner
incoming a new chapter.

## Nursing Rhyme
### after Lemn Sissay

I like stories with cups of coffee,
Fresh scrubs and a side of cake
I like a challenge but you know - deeply,
I like veins the size of a rake.
I like fluid lines with no kink,
Questions that make me think
Machines that don't beep so much,
The miracle of the human touch.

I like mitered corners on a bed
Bandages wrapped around tiny heads
I like steady flowing drips,
Breakfasts after night shifts
I like soft shoes on my feet
I like neat handover sheets
I like dressings that really stick,
Smooth on all corners, that's just slick!

I like crocs with quirky socks,
Therapy dogs with curly locks
A healed wound is an amen!
Also, doctors with their own pens.
I like being a ray of hope
The lubb-dubb through a stethoscope
I like helping those in need
Handwriting that I can read.

I like cards that say thank you,
Sometimes a sweet or two
I like big bright smiles
That make this job worthwhile.
I like how strong we are inside
When faced with things we cannot hide.
Just a few things I like, spattered in verse
The small delights of being a nurse.

## Coffee Rounds

Flat white, latte, white americano,
Coconut flat white, soya cappuccino,
Mocha, cortado, caramel macchiato,
Flat black, double shot of espresso.

Then there's those strong enough
to do this job with just hot chocolate,
Or herbal tea, or would you believe - decaf?
The audacity of all of it!

Jim once asked me to reveal the holy secret,
Of coping with the intensity that comes along with it.
The recipe is simple: first, coffee - a lot of it,
And then as needed, a good cry in the toilet.

## Departure Gate

The gates towered upon us and
intimidated our separation anxiety.
If the saddest part of the ship is the stern,
then this is the stern that I face to overcome.

A ginger man with a sleeve tattoo
once told me that I
was brave for moving to a place
where no one knew me.

Only when I found myself marching
through the departure gates
without looking back
at the ones who loved me,
necklaced with tears,
did I really understand
     what he was trying to say.

## Agatha

Dear sweet Agatha,
please grant me the strength
To survive this long shift
until the very end!
Grant healing to my patients
even as they sleep
Give me compassion and caring hands,
strong legs and bouncy feet.
We may not be regal
or worthy of a crown,
But hand us wit and humour
albeit faced with a code brown.
May we have courage nothing short of mythical
to stand by those waiting for a miracle.
Oh sweet, holy Agatha,
keep us away from harm and bane
So come morning we can get up,
and do this all again.

II.

"How we spend our days is, of course, how we spend our lives. - Annie Dillard

## Night Shift

A hundred and twenty two minutes, / and the siren blared on / like there was nothing left to lose.

In his delirium, / someone pushed / the fire alarm button, / smashed it like his last hope, / ran to the lobby / and is now in stand-off / with the security team.

Headaches hummed for those / who just had their heads opened. / No hope of an override switch, / when the fire seal is broken / by a push.

I clutched the phone with both hands - / pressed it tight against my right ear.

This time - / there was no understanding / laced in the voice / of the man from the fire department. / "If the patient calls us again we have to respond / even if it is a false alarm." / "Lock her phone if you have to."

A voice howled along the corridor: / "They are lying to us! / The firemen are coming, do not worry!"

As if on cue - / three call lights twinkled in unison, / summoning a beep I know so well /that I hear it in my sleep.

I gazed around / like a soldier needing a strategy. / Cleared my throat and / aimed my eyes at the clock;

It was only five past ten.

## Homecoming

The titanium plate in your head / was only about three months old / when your eyes / followed your mother's figure / as she rushed, / and slipped backside first / on the white feathery rug.

Your laughter rippled / from mid-air /and into her heart that had missed you / long enough for yearning / to turn itself / into a gentle mourn.

For you have not laughed, / or smiled, / or walked, / or talked, / since the day your skull broke apiece.

This metal chair / became an extension of you; / here but not quite yourself.

Who knew that eternity / could last five seconds long? / She exhaled joy, / hands cupped on trembling lips, / her laughter swirled with yours / to celebrate / the unspeakable gladness / of welcoming you.

Remember when you were once so lost / deep into this body, / but somewhere into the haze of your being, / you fought your way back home? / And darling - welcome home.

## Shattered

From where I was, it may well have been,
a small blast of confetti in suspended animation.
It could sit on the palm of my hand,
    ready to be kissed away,
like wisps of dandelion on a windy, blue May.

Except, instead of birthday sprinkles,
    it was all black and white.
Except, instead of a party,
    it was a scan of your face.
Fragments of you shattered into shrapnel,
Echoes of where his fists landed
      again
           and again
              and again.
Under swollen lips, you mumbled,
    "Leaving him is not the hard part,
          I've done it many times."

The CAT scanner bared your bones
    but not your spirit.
Underneath crushed bone,
you are not broken where it counts.
And from there, one day,
may you find it in you
    to sprint without turning back,
To pack your bags together with
    all the reasons that kept you
from letting go of the man
who's greatest kindness in this life
was knocking you out cold.

## Walking With Sue

A sheet of paper waved  from my right.
"Do you know where this is?"
She said to no one in particular,
but my reflexes, - of course,
lured me to answer.

> Eyebrows met in worry,
> Breathing sharp and short from rushing,
> Beads of sweat across her forehead.
> "Should I walk you there?"
> "Oh, would you mind?"
> Truth is,
> I was not going that way,
> but today, I had time.

Layers of clothing hung from her frame,
Her walk - a shuffle more than a stride.
Bony hands and sunken cheeks,
Dry, wiry hair rocking from side to side.
For a mere two minutes,
she compressed her battle for months:
Once upon a failing liver,
followed by an infection that she thought
was the end of her.
And yet-
She walked out of intensive care
just four weeks ago...
Her fight took her to this day -
her first chemotherapy.

I dropped her off and really meant it
when I wished her good luck.
She grinned and faced me with
    ocean eyes,
"Thanks for the company, call me Sue."
Like I was some newfound friend.

Her exhaustion failed to hide
who she was today,
One storm of a woman
not ready to give up just yet.

## Disfiguring

Nurse, can you see this?
~~My hideous jaw and long face.~~
~~I've been hurting since someone called me ugly,~~
~~I was seven years old, dancing on stage.~~
~~I hide from the mirror because all I can see~~
~~is how broken I am and my crooked front teeth.~~
~~This spot that none of my friends can find?~~
~~I rubbed it for nine hours~~
~~Until it started to bleed.~~

Please don't think I am insane.
~~Maybe I am.~~

I could not see what your eyes
kept showing you every day
But I am here, and I heard it all
All the words you did not say.

# Memory

On mornings of clarity,
you would tell me about your life.
Your sons -
    how they cried,
because you started calling out their names
    while you were all sat around for dinner.
You grew up on a coffee plantation,
    with a father who showed you hard work
    and a passion for caffeine.

You lost your mind every day,
though by the morning you came back.
You fear the day it carries you away for good,
turning your memory into black

So on mornings of clarity,
        we'd sit and have a talk,
So that someone else can remember
who you are long after things are not the same;
When the bandit comes and gets you,
Leaving nothing behind,
        nothing but your children's names.

## Bright Yellow Bag

She entered the room
    with her bright yellow bag,
Plopped it onto the chair,
then bounced in front of them
like an unbeaten force
something keeps trying to stop.

She felt the need to say -
"I have not felt this happy in a very long time."
They paused -
because they knew how much
that really meant.
As if the cancer was not enough,
the radiation
eroded the good parts left of her.

We are all but countdowns
trying to get through and thrive,
But how often do we forget that
we're not making it out of here alive?
So be strong, be kind,
    cherish victories - big or small
Wave your hope like a flag.
As bright as the hope she carried with her,
in her bright yellow bag.

## Widower

He broke down like a pile of bones,
 - bare, exposed, unprotected.
The moment he said
      he just missed her so much,
All that was left was a man further wilted
by forty years of love vaporised by a second.
I swallowed the globe
climbing the attic of my throat,
Looked for words but found nothing
      until the air had cleared.
Perhaps silence is the correct answer,
when time remains as the only cure
for the pain this life comes promised with;
      and here we are all but trying to endure.

## Metastasis

It's terminal -
> the black magic had pranced from
> your kidneys to your lungs,
> to your fractured jaw that split
> from the power of this malignant force.

It's terminal -
> the doctors said there was nothing they can do.
> Three weeks ago, you heard the news,
> your daughter lost her battle with it too.

The war is over, defeat is here
There's one last mission left in you:
Lay your child to rest just right before
the final funeral you'll ever have to go to.

## Homeless

Nurse, I am sorry but I have no address,
Four years fought to live another day
And still there are times when this life feels like,
nothing but a slow decay.

Nurse, can you show them how you look past
these dirty hands and bristly face?
To ignore the stench I have long gotten used to,
and treat me with an ounce of grace.

Nurse, do you think they will help me?
I have tried hard not to get here so-
Tell them this filth is the only thing criminal about me,
Tell them I am not lost, I just have nowhere to go.

## Christmas Card

Scribbled in child's handwriting,
the card read,

Joan,my darling you are always
laughing. Have a good name
but always smile for me
Love,
Stephen M

your heart -
  indelible to the tumour
that left you scrambling
        for your daughter's name,
        countless times in a day.
left you learning how to write again,
left you tracing your steps like a wandering babe.

You wrestled the pen -
A slanted J, a wobbly O
the crooked  A and a wavy N.
These misshapen letters
    will always and truly be,
the sweetest version of thank you
someone has ever given me.

## Paula's Crater

when you fell on your head,
it was a trauma call not so major
but there was so much blood,
it trailed on your face
like it came from an overhead shower.

the wound at the back of your head
- a Rafflesia.
broken skin gaped open like
a surprised mouth,
erupted scalp with frayed fleshy edges,
skull exposed in the heart of jagged tissue.

we became friends for seven weeks,
you turned seventy a month ago
but always stared back as the formidable
twenty - year - old you have always been.
the crater sealed to a bald spot
the size of a coin.
after weeks of loving care,
you smiled and turned around,
made me laugh with your plans
        of getting pink hair.

Before leaving, you handed over
 a tiny box with three glass angels,
        the size of thumbs.
"I usually bite but thank goodness
        you have a gentle touch"
May these angels remind you of what you are,
So long, don't miss me too much."

## Losing Sight

Never-mind the rude doctor who
asked if we were done with this room
without as much as a glance
        or a fake hello.

Alcohol is the poison you drowned this life in,
because your reality looked better in a blur.
Even if it shrunk you to a corner,
where you cower as shy children do.

If only you could remember what hit you that day-
But the bottle had erased more than you would like,
And now there is only darkness on that left side.
The void strangely worse than the cloud
        in the same way silence is painfully loud.

I wondered if you can feel the teardrop
        growing from the corner of the night
of that plucked eyeball.

## Terminal

Chances are, I will be gone,
by the time you get to sit and hear
these words I wished I knew before,
all my time walked out the door.

Chances are, we'll both be grieving
the time we lost and won't be sharing,
So listen and take my advice to heart,
Keep it close and do not be afraid to start.

Your real life is with friends and family,
and never with the people at work.
So do not miss a birthday party
just so your boss won't go berserk.

Travel far and travel wide,
Remember that pain tends to subside,
Climb a mountain, feel the rain
Love deeply, love insane.

Tear your eyes away from the screen,
Go outside and enjoy the scene.
Jump on your bed, dance in the kitchen
Make happiness your life mission

Tell that boy next door you love him
Take your chances in romance.
And of course, go get a dog,
Whenever you get the chance.

I beg you, fear not when I'm no longer here,
For I am mere stardust returned to the air.
My love for you shall never stop,
Although for now, my time is up.

III.

"Courage is grace under pressure".
- Ernest Hemingway

## Final Shift
### after Ocean Vuong

*Two babies and 12 mothers and nurses were killed in a militant attack on a hospital in the Afghan capital Kabul on Tuesday morning. - BBC News, May 12, 2020.*

It rained when you were born;
but not like what you'd think.
I wish I could tell you the skies
rejoiced with rain,
instead of these hailing
bullets that gave an answer
to some angry man's scream.

Red carpet made from blood
  of mothers and newborns
    swerved across the floor,
    like some
highway from hell that's found
its way to worldly things.

A figure in the corner of my eye -
Hunched over, swimming in red,
her body caved into a shield,
hugged the life she just brought here,
when the aimed rifle spat a single bullet
that ended two lives.

A creeping pool of crimson
    crowned your bassinet,
The sink we first washed you in,
    now spattered in red.
Pockmarks on the wall, a quivering trail
    of what the devil has left.

Is anyone ever made to get past this?
Should I bleed to death and never get to find out
    then I am lucky for sure-
to be spared of moving on from something
that will kill me countless times over,
long after these exit wounds have dried into scars.

*May 12, 2020 was International Nurses Day.*

## Your Heroine

When the invisible foe stirred into the air,
cutting breaths,
taking bodies,
infesting our peace,
You looked upon me and saw a hero
for the things I do every day.

My unappreciated toil never ceased to exist -
I have held motherless newborns,
witnessed inglorious ends
that came with sudden demise,
cried with men unprepared in the face of death,
long before the air became sinister.

The fear in my chest burns
like hot breath,
moving out and in again
against this tight mask;
like heartache when someone loses a fight.

With the same heart, I praise
those who endure.
Now I know that war-zones take place
albeit missing of bullets and bombs,
Leaving behind a trail of bodies
Some of them with faces I know.
Can we ever thank the brave enough
for giving the villain a good fight?

Hail the unsung hero who is remembered
Only when tragedies strike
        and times go forlorn.
When all the passion is spent
and there is nothing left to spare,
I will take a gentle bow,
And think of my little one at home
        left unhugged.
If only I could buy that doll she cried for
with these rounds of applause.

## Portrait

This face is a ghost of the ruins
no one will find buried in the years to come.

Come brush this tousled hair,
Witness these chapped lips.

Unveil my purple skin,
Marked and cracked by this mask
that suffocates in order to protect.

Run your fingers along the ridges it
made on these cheeks,
Feel where it sliced across my flesh.

And formed dry river beds
That guide streaming tears.

Watch these blisters flare
like angry little fires.

This face is the map of ground zero,
Man down, man down!

Down went the hero.

## OFW

*dedicated to Kenneth Lambatan (1986-2020)*
*A son, a friend, a nurse.*

My last breath was the antithesis
    of a young, vibrant life.
Last goodbyes said over bright screens
that crossed oceans for miles,
The anguish of a mother
    surviving her son,
Is this all that is left for us?
Tears shed over plastic and glass.
It's hard to name anything
    we would not give,
to rethink the dream that took us here.
Just sing me that song again,
let that voice soothe me
    nice and slow,
A lullaby sending me to sleep,
    as this body fails me and lets go.
Ashen skin against latex glove,
melodies crooned over the distance,
The flat line on that monitor,
    an exit of my existence.

## Epitaph

May you look at this and remember,
If history fails to write us in the slight,
That once - we were fathers, sons, daughters and wives
Who walked with fear but carried on,
Until we paid dearly with our lives.

# FLORENCE

From this point forward,
  Let it be known,
    Our spirits never faltered or
      Ran out of ways to get back up
        Even after when some man said,
          Now is not the time to talk about the worth of
                                        nurses.
            Can he realize how wrong he is, if he finds himself
            Exhaling to a respirator, nursed by the very
                                people he chose to forget?

## Priceless

It's a calling - a vocation, you said.
Because it takes someone to see the joy
              -or sense
in what I do.

You mistook my blue uniform for an ocean
to drown my lived experience.
So you can brand it as charity,
because who can deny
how it all fits so well?

I watched a man at the mercy
of the breathing end of a respirator,
Watched him shrink to a pile of dead flowers,
until he crumbled into something
no one he loved could recognize.

I watched people bid farewell,
through plastic screens
that I held with aching arms.
Because how long is long enough when
faced with the last goodbye?

If you want to, I can tell you
what real fear looks like,
it looks quiet and stops time,
it grips your throat so you don't scream,
it makes you hear through someone's eyes.

This year was the year
of the nurse and I can tell you,
I killed my alarm
four, five times so I can wake up to
A job that's starting to feel like it
      loathes me.

In case you did not see it,
this year of the nurse,
fear ate me but I went out there anyway.

A nurse my age died so I
thought about my own death
more times than I would like.

I watched parents leave their children,
Tucked themselves into hotels because
sometimes safety looks like separation.

I pushed my anxiety aside because my badge
     read 'Nurse'
And the world said it needed me.

Someone once told me
I am worth my weight in gold.
I went ahead and asked whatever this meant to you,
and in so many goddamn words you said -

"Nothing."

## Aftermath

They say it's supposed
to look pretty,
Maybe pink -
      with tea light candles,
bath salts and a lot of lathered soap.

Nobody tells you what coping looks like,
when it takes on the form of a damp spirit.
A reflection in the mirror
      far from familiar.
When it's sleeping in your scrubs
when you know you shouldn't.
Waking up in the middle of the night
to eat a cold sandwich sat on the counter.
The one you looked forward to having
in front of the sink,
      yesterday.

It's standing under a blast of angry water,
feel it pelting against your back, your hair.
It's staring at a blank wall
wishing you can wring your heart out
To make space,
so you can drench it more.

This shift is over but why
      does the rest of this life
feel like an aftermath
      rather than a harbour?

Let me tell you something
nursing school never taught me:

We -
we are not perfect but
we are too good for this world.

You -
you are worth more
than the pay rise they refuse you.

You-
you deserve more than an applause.

You-
and I mean no one else but you.

You are the kind mercy
this world counts on to continue,
Unlike mean men in suits who
keep the weak on their knees -

You are magnanimous.

## Bravo

So let me tell you something,
In case you were too blind to see,
Or turned deaf like when we said,
"We need more PPE."

While you were out there clapping,
You thought you saw people bowing their heads.
This is our life, not a curtain call,
They were not bowing, they were dropping dead.

## Farewell Note

As if this life is not short enough,
a thief now looms to cut
this moment of a lifetime
to a spark no one else will celebrate
but the two of us,
because we smell like
      home to each other.

If this crook takes my body now,
and I am not here when you turn eighty,
If this crook withers me to nothing before
I get to say I love you a million times - I'm sorry.
If in forty, fifty years I am not there to say -
"Look baby we made it."
Know that I would have rather stayed,
and frayed, and greyed,
and turn silver with you.
Watch the sun set on us,
our veins drained from our youth.

When your skin has turned into
      soft wrinkled peaks,
And you miss how your shoulders
      cradle my round jelly cheeks,
On a clear night, my darling -
      open your hand into the air,
And by firefly or by stardust, I promise
I will be there.

♦♦♦♦

"We write from life and call it literature, and literature lives
because we are in it."
— F. Sionil José, In Search of the Word: Selected Essays

# ABOUT THE AUTHOR

Joan Cruz graduated Bachelor of Science in Nursing last 2009 in the Philippines under a full scholarship. She worked in various specialities before moving to the UK to work for the National Health Service in 2014. She was a Junior Sister in Neuroscience before taking on her current post as Clinical Nurse Specialist for Oral and Maxillofacial Surgery at Kings College Hospital NHS Foundation Trust. She lives in Northfleet, looks after twenty something fish babies and is a self confessed plant mom.

Printed in Great Britain
by Amazon